Ronald M. Lawrence, M.D.

Goodbye Pain!

Two Dozen Ways To Prevent Pain

Also Featuring:

The CICO Diet Plan

*(Because weight control and
good nutrition help to control pain!)*

Published by

Woodbridge Press
Santa Barbara, California

Published and distributed by

Woodbridge Press Publishing Company
Post Office Box 6189
Santa Barbara, California 93160

Distributed simultaneously in the United States and Canada

Printed in the United States of America

Library of Congress Cataloging-in-Publication data

Lawrence, Ronald Melvin, 1926–
    Goodbye pain!

    1. Pain—Prevention—Popular works.   2. Pain—Popular
works.   I. Title.
RB127.L32   1988   616'.0472   88-28001
ISBN 0-88007-169-9

Photography: Kevin Stapleton
Model: Anne Stapleton in most photographs

The Author

Ronald M. Lawrence, M.D., Ph.D., is a founding member of the International Association for the Study of Pain, a former member of The President's National Advisory Council on Aging, a member of the Advisory Board of the Alcoholism, Drug Abuse, and Mental Health Administration, and a Medical Advisor to The President's Council on Physical Fitness and Sport. An Assistant Clinical Professor, Neuropsychiatric Institute, School of Medicine, University of California at Los Angeles, he is a diplomate of the American National Board of Psychiatry, the American Board of Orthopedic and Neurologic Surgeons, and the American Board of Electroencephalography. He has for 35 years been engaged in medical practice in North Hollywood and Agoura, California.

He has served as guest lecturer at Harvard University, Yale University, University of California, Tulane University, and others. He holds numerous fellowships and memberships and is the author of 25 scientific papers in the fields of Pain, Neurophysiology, Cerebral Blood Flow, Electroencephalography, Sports Psychology, and Neurology.

He holds or has held positions as President, American Medical Athletic Association; President and Founder, American Medical Joggers Association; Director, National Jogging Association; Consultant, U.S. Olympic Committee; President, Acupuncture Medical Association of America; President, American Academy of Acupuncture Medicine; Secretary, American Academy of Sports Physicians; Director, American Technion Society; and others.

Among his awards are the Philip Noel Baker Research Award, United Nations (UNESCO), presented at the Montreal Olympics; Maimonides Award, American Technion Society; Peace Medal, Technion Medical School, Haifa, Israel; Research Associate, Rockefeller Institute for Medical Research, New York.

Contents

Foreword: *How to Get the Help You Need from This Book*

The need for this book has been on my mind for many years—but a busy medical practice is not conducive to writing! With the publication of an article on the prevention of pain in the *National Enquirer*—based on my work—and many such articles in other publications, I realized how important it was to produce such a book; many people obviously are interested in pain relief—because they need it!

In more than 35 years of medical practice, I have attended more than 150,000 patients, and the vast majority of these people had pain problems, most of which could have been prevented by observing some basic considerations. Many of these considerations are so simple that it seems a pity to be unaware of them.

Numerous books have been written on attempting to control chronic pain once it develops, but books on how to actually stop the evolution of chronic pain are rare.

Many of the concepts I present in this book have never before been written about. I learned them the hard way, by studying my patients carefully over many years. This is why I am dedicating this book to my patients—without them, I could never have developed the information which I now pass on to you.

Please read this book carefully; it has purposely been kept simple so that you won't have to spend much time in absorbing the information. I suggest that you peruse the book quickly—all at one time, and then read each section slowly. Even more important, study the photographs in detail. I chose the pictures with great concentration and care. The photographs are essentially the heart of the book, since you can learn almost all there is to know about pain prevention by grasping the simple facts conveyed in each picture. As the Chinese say, "One picture is worth a thousand words," and that certainly applies here. Don't try to fully absorb the entire book in one day—take it a little at a time, one section each day. In that way, you will "digest" it better, and the information will stay with you for a pain-free lifetime.

If possible, try to obtain my other books, although they are not essential to your reading this one. You can get more detailed information on certain aspects of diet, exercise, massage, and disease prevention from the works listed at the back of this book. Additionally, I have included two chapters on special new dieting aids for those of you who have to lose weight—excess weight is a major contributor to the problems of pain. Even those of us who are satisfied with our weight must be on guard against putting on unwanted, unhealthy pounds.

Part I

Proven Ways to Prevent Pain

Two Dozen Ways to Prevent or Relieve Pain

Most chronic pain is self-inflicted! That is my professional opinion after nearly four decades of treating people in pain. By self-inflicted, I mean the bloodless, bodily harm we do ourselves by some of the simple, but injurious, habits and activities of daily living.

The most routine act, such as sitting in a chair and watching television, can be the cause of lifetime pain. Even the clothes you wear, the way you eat, the way you sleep, and the bed you sleep on can be sources of chronic pain.

As a neurologist, I specialize in the treatment of pain. As a former member of The President's National Advisory Council on Aging, I observed on a wide scale the problems of long-term pain, experienced especially by older people. As a president of the American Medical Athletic Association and secretary of the American Academy of Sports Physicians, I have become intimately familiar with the connection between physical activity and pain among people of all ages.

You, too, can become more aware of the effects many of your activities and lifestyle modes have on your body—*and probably prevent a full 80 percent of the pain you might otherwise suffer!*

There is much more you can do for chronic pain than "learning to live with it," or becoming an aspirin addict. In this book are more than two dozen ideas that have helped my patients to prevent pain problems and to ease those already present. Hopefully, they can help you as well!

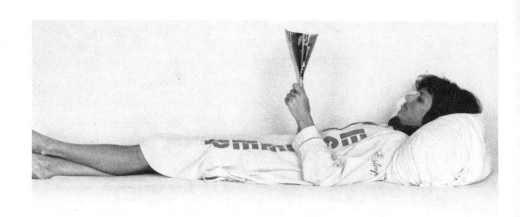

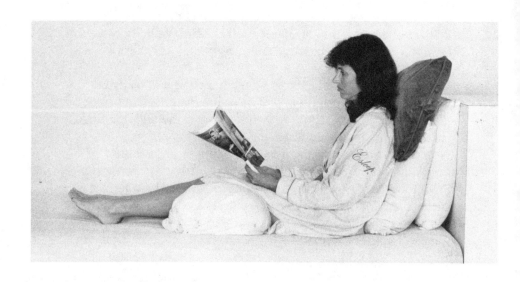

14

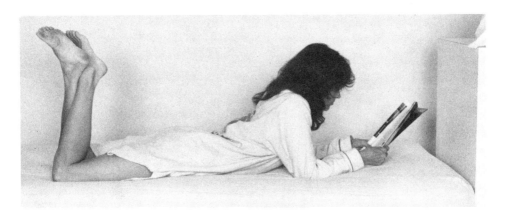

Reading Can Be a Headache

Headache is one of the most common chronic pain problems, and it is frequently attributed to some exotic or ominous cause. More often than not, however, the cause is some simple habit of everyday living.

One largely unsuspected, but leading, cause is reading in bed. Lack of proper pillow support, with the neck bent at too sharp an angle, is an open invitation to trouble. This unnatural position strains the muscles attached to the back of the skull and initiates a painful cycle of muscular tension, neckaches, and headaches. Over a long period of time, it contributes to degenerative changes in the neck vertebrae, resulting in arthritic pain.

If you insist on reading in bed, prop yourself up as if *sitting in a chair*. Also make sure you place a pillow under your knees. Keeping your legs straight in front of you puts stress on your lower back muscles. Lying on your abdomen (as shown in the photograph) and holding a book can be comfortable for a few minutes, but when this position is held for more than just a few minutes, it leads to marked neck and back strain as well as stress in the shoulder areas.

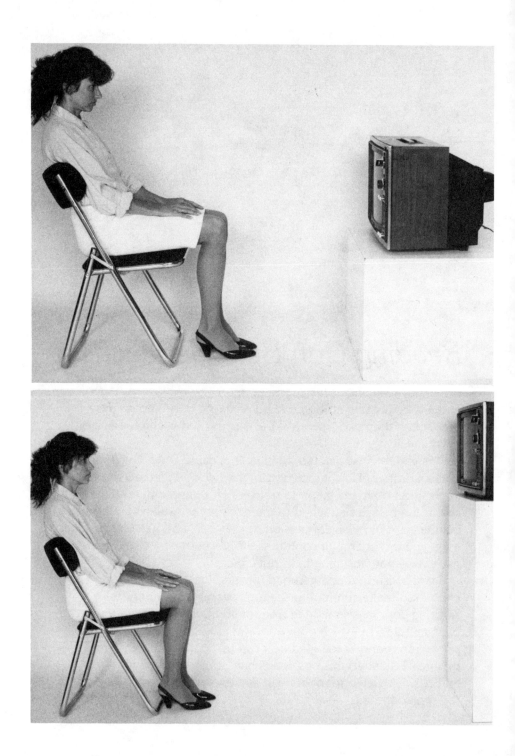

Make Light of Eyestrain

Eyestrain leads to headaches. Always read in a good light. If the lighting is poor, you can cause or worsen the condition called astigmatism. In astigmatism, there is an imbalance of the intrinsic eye muscles, which can lead to headaches and blurred vision.

Watching television with head and eyes at an angle can also cause eyestrain, astigmatism, and headaches. A torsion created in the neck can reduce circulation to the head by "kinking" arteries in the neck. Headaches may then develop, as well as blurring of vision, due to changes in blood flow.

An average size television set should be located no less than four to six feet away and directly in your normal line of vision, or perhaps slightly above the line of vision.

We tend to think that the lighting from an average ceiling fixture is enough to read by, but in many cases this is not true. Certainly, it is better to have a reading lamp close by. The light should be directed over your shoulder onto the book, magazine, or newspaper you are reading. The glare on the page from this light should be as little as possible. Modern fluorescent lighting can be very effective if the fixture is working properly. If there is a flickering, due to a damaged bulb or to an impaired starter, one can develop marked eyestrain problems.

Tension Headaches

Stress on the neck muscles, due to postural improprieties or muscular strain, is one of the most common causes of the headaches frequently referred to as "tension headaches," or muscle contraction headaches.

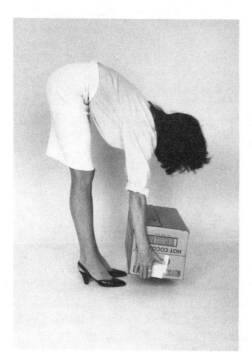

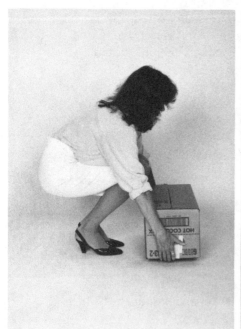

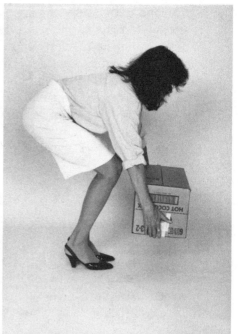

Easing Your Aching Back

Lower back pain is probably the most common complaint among my patients. The most frequent cause is improper lifting. You can stay out of trouble if you remember to use *all of you* when lifting. That means using your arms, body, and legs. Most people tend to just bend down and lift with their arms. This strains the lower back muscles and vertebral joints, often leading quickly to muscular aches. Keep that up and you will be contributing to the eventual development of degenerative spinal arthritis and additional chronic pain.

It is not the weight of the object that does the damage; it is the way you lift. No matter how light an object appears to be, you should bend at the knees, gently go into a squat position, and then lift with your entire body. As you lift, try not to twist from one side of your body to the other. Such rotary motion causes a lot of back problems, particularly in the workplace. Always try to turn your entire body when lifting, distributing the weight equally between both arms.

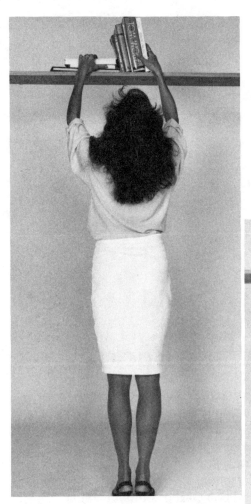

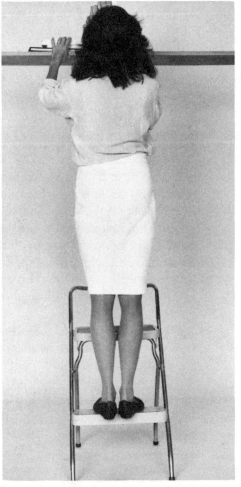

Avoiding a Pain in the Neck

Neck pain is the third most common chronic pain problem—after lower back pain and headache. As we get older, sudden movements of the neck can damage ligaments, muscles, and bone and promote the development of chronic pain.

Even the simple motion of looking upward can be risky. I usually recommend that patients past age 40 do not look upward unless they absolutely have to. Tasks such as changing a light bulb or getting something off a high shelf should be performed while using a small step stool or ladder. Keep your head in as neutral a position as possible. In extending the neck, such as in an upward gaze, older persons may have a tendency to get very dizzy. This can result in a fall, which might fracture a hip or other part of the body.

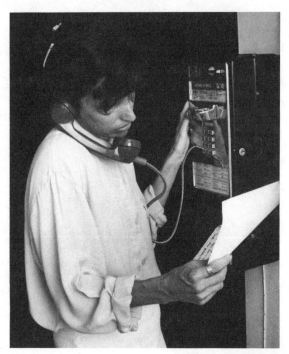

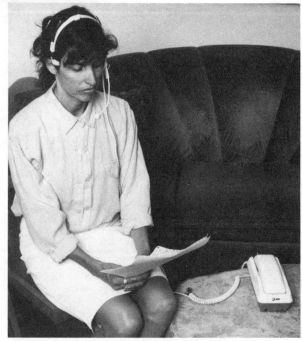

Telephones Can Ring in Pain

The telephone is probably a necessity in your life, but if you're not careful, it can become a *real* pain-in-the-neck. A frequent cause of neck pain today is the habit of tilting the head to one side or the other in order to hold the telephone receiver against a shoulder while doing other things with the hands. It is a bad habit, and it can cause severe neck strain and pain.

If you need free hands while "on the phone," use a headset. These sets can be rented inexpensively from your local telephone company, or they can be purchased for under $25 from many radio and gadget supply houses. If you spend many hours a day on the telephone, this small expenditure is certainly worth it. As a bonus, the sound is usually improved, too, because of better contact between the receiver and the ear. Can you imagine the telephone operator cocking a telephone receiver between her shoulder and ear?

Parents may not realize it, but their children are well on their way to developing chronic inflammatory changes in the neck area if they are using the telephone in an improper manner. I see many men and women in their early twenties who have already developed arthritic changes or calcific deposits in the neck because of this very poor habit.

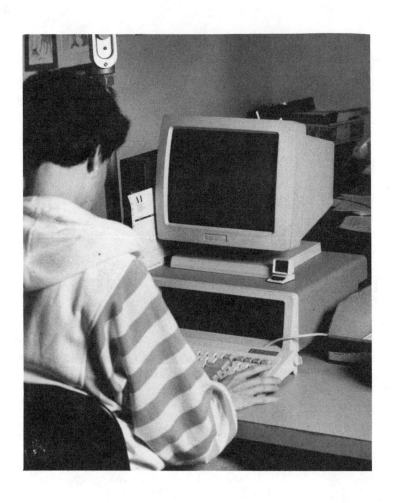

Work Posture Can Cause Pain

Another common cause of eyestrain and neck problems, as well as shoulder and upper back pain, is the improper use of computer screens—increasingly prevalent in office settings. The computer or word processor operator should comply with all the suggestions I have made elsewhere about standing up periodically and stretching and walking about. Additionally, the computer screen should be at eye level so the neck is not bent either upward or downward in order for the operator to view the screen properly.

In the photograph, you will notice that the operator has to flex the neck and head forward in order to read the screen. This is not a satisfactory work position. In this case the screen should be elevated slightly.

Another problem lies with the keyboard, which should be—as with typewriters—at a level at which the arms and elbows can be held in a stress-free position.

Neglect of these warnings will lead to all sorts of chronic pain problems in the future. Eyestrain does occur, when viewing such screens, as is now well known, and it is important for the worker to determine whether such eyestrain exists. If so, it should be brought to the attention of the employer, since long-term tolerance of an uncomfortable working situation will lead to trouble not only for the worker but for the employer as well.

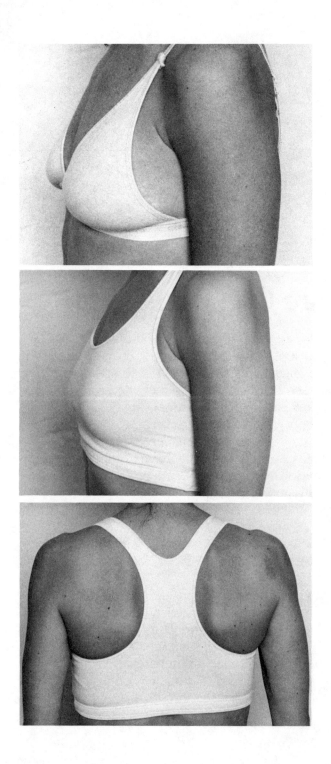

Breast Support

An active woman needs proper support for her breasts, especially if she is large-breasted. I recommend a well-constructed sports bra for large-breasted women who run or jog. This prevents bouncing of the breasts and damage to the Cooper's ligament, the connection between the breasts and the chest wall. I have treated many women who suffer from pain just because they prefer a natural, braless look when exercising.

Actually, large-breasted women should *always* wear a sturdy bra. Regularly going braless or wearing a flimsy bra, can lead to sagging breasts and a condition called kyphosis—an unsightly humped back. This is more likely to happen to large-breasted women than they realize. Not only does it look bad, it is painful, too. Kyphosis can be accompanied by arthritic changes in the upper back, neck, and shoulders. Pain can commence in the upper back while a woman is in her mid-twenties and peak to an intolerable level by age 40. Some large-breasted women who are sensitive about their breast size tend to pull in their breasts and hunch up. This will also lead to kyphosis and pain.

Everyday bras should have wide, solid shoulder straps. Reserve the narrow-strap models for dates or special occasions when you are wearing a low-cut dress. Narrow straps can cause chronic pain because the straps cut into the trapezius muscles, which lie between the shoulder and neck. Irritation of a major nerve, the suprascapular, can occur as well, since it is located in this area. The straps can cut off the blood supply to the trapezius muscle, and this is painful as well. Straps should be at least an inch wide for women with large—or even average-size breasts. It is also important that bras have a solid, padded lower band.

Tread Lightly to Avoid Pain

Walking or jogging on hard surfaces is an invitation to degenerative arthritis. The human body does not seem to be made for ambulation on concrete or other hard surfaces. Each time you plant your foot on such a surface, you deliver a force throughout your body equal to two and one-half times your weight. The spinal column absorbs much of this jolt, and eventually a painful osteoarthritis condition may develop along the spine. Avoid those hard surfaces as much as you can. Do your walking on softer surfaces, and if you have to jog, it is even better to jog or run on flat, grassy strips or on dirt trails.

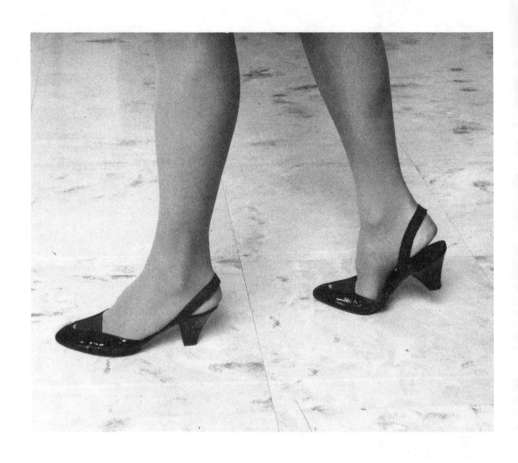

Shopping for Trouble

Walking in shopping malls is particularly difficult, although you may not realize it while you are doing it. Have you ever noticed how tired you feel after a day of shopping in such a mall? It is difficult to obtain traction on the smooth, glossy floor surfaces that are in most shopping centers. If you cannot get proper traction, you must use your entire lower extremity to move; and, in fact, you are using your entire body in a stressful fashion to propel yourself over such a smooth surface. For such occasions, it is best to wear shoes that will provide good traction. The average walking or running shoe should be very good.

Now that grandma and grandpa, as well as many other citizens, have joined the mall walkers, we are seeing thousands of people using these areas for exercise. This is a very good thing! However, take a lesson from grandma and grandpa and notice how many of them have purchased shoes that will provide traction for walking in the mall!

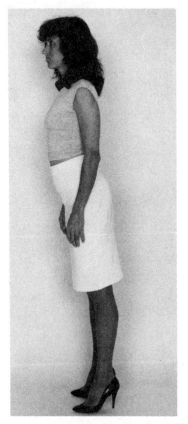

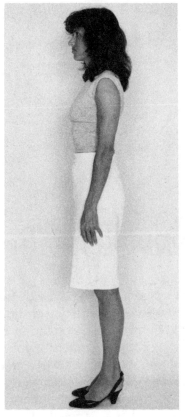

Good Heels—No Pain

High heels mean high risk for lower back pain. They increase the natural curve of the lower spine, stressing the muscles in that area. Regular wearing of high-heeled shoes can cause arthritis and chronic strain in the back as well. Neurologists and orthopedists treat many women for lower back pain caused by years of everyday wearing of high heels. Use them only for social occasions, or at work if you usually work sitting down with very little standing or walking. If you must wear heels, you can use a low-cut heel.

Remember also to use a firm heel counter (at the back of the shoe) to prevent your heels from sliding from side to side. This can occur with women's shoes that use a flimsy strap or straps for heel stabilization. A good heel cup that keeps the foot from sliding and a good arch support are very important.

You will notice that in the photograph, there is a marked increase in the low back curve of the model wearing the high heels. When she changes to the lower heels, you see a much more natural and gentle curve in the low back.

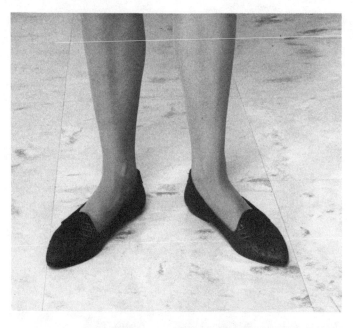

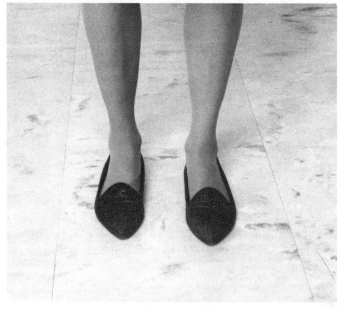

Pains that Shoes Can Cure

Knee problems are common in this country, and a major cause is improper footwear. The feet tend to splay outward (a condition known as pronation), putting extra stress on the knees. In time, this stress leads to the development of arthritis. You should wear shoes that tend to keep your feet pointing in a relatively straight line as you walk, or even as you stand. The American Indians walked with their big toes more or less in a straight line with the heels, and they were noted for their ability to walk long distances without great fatigue. We can all take a lesson from these native Americans.

I particularly recommend an inexpensive longitudinal arch to be placed in your shoes. In most instances, it will solve the problem. Such an arch tends to reduce the amount of pronation many of us have.

If you are a runner, it is wise to be especially wary of problems caused by out-turned feet. Many runners I have seen over many years develop knee, hip, and back problems (and even occasionally neck and shoulder problems) due to pronation of the feet. Those of us born flat-footed (and I am not alluding to our police friends) have a propensity to develop splayed feet. A simple arch correction can, in most cases, help us a great deal.

Your family doctor or neighborhood podiatrist can offer help with foot problems.

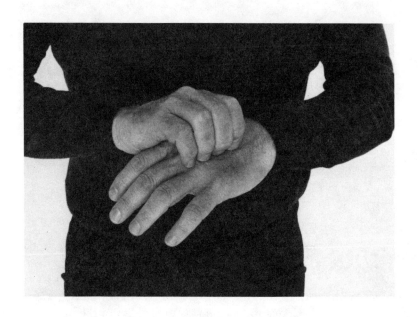

A Helping Hand Massage

While we are dealing with our lower appendages, let us consider the upper ones as well. As we age, arthritis frequently develops in our hands. It is a consequence of the aging process and also of improper use of our hands over many years. Take a few moments out of each day to massage your hands. If you do this regularly, you can increase the blood circulation, helping to diminish the degenerating processes as well as relieving some of the ligament tension. This will significantly cut the potential for pain.

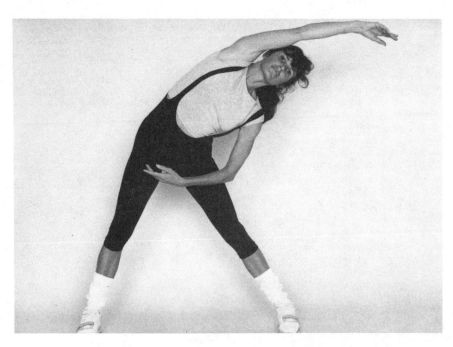

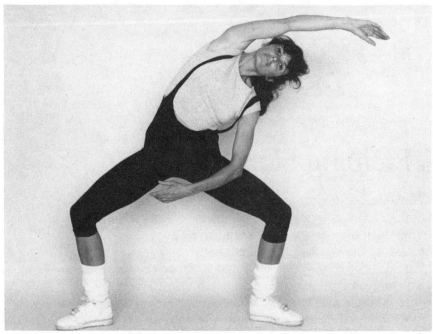

Pain-Free Exercise

Many women (and men, too) are developing chronic pain problems by plunging into those popular videotape exercise programs with too much zeal and not enough common sense. Trying to do too much too soon is a sure way to overstrain muscles and cause yourself pain. Jane Fonda didn't become a whiz at her routine overnight; she built up to it slowly.

Not only can you cause chronic pain, but you can also put yourself out of commission permanently through improper exercise. Torn ligaments, tendons, and muscles are not pleasant to live with. Always start out slowly and cautiously when exercising. Remember that preliminary flexibility exercises are vital to the prevention of such problems. At the back of this book is a list of recommended literature dealing, among other things, with stretching. Taking a few moments to stretch before exercising is a very wise precaution.

Remember that exercising with your knees straight will place a strain on your back, and you should not do that until you are well on in your program. This may take months to accomplish. Notice also, from the photographs, the importance of keeping your back in a neutral position when doing certain types of bends or stretches.

Watching some people do these aerobic exercises reminds me of early circus days when "India rubber men" did their fanciful contortions. However, few of us can emulate them, and trying to do so will result in a circus of horrors from which there is no escape!

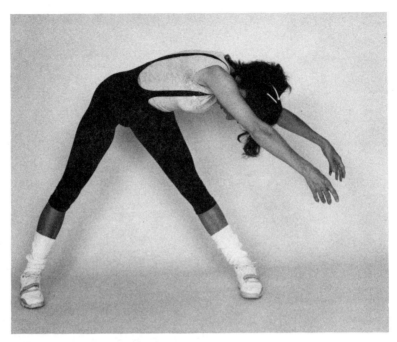

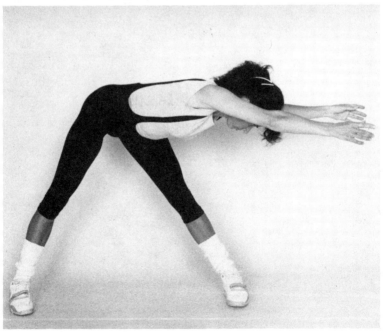

Goodbye Pain! 41

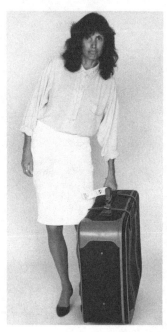

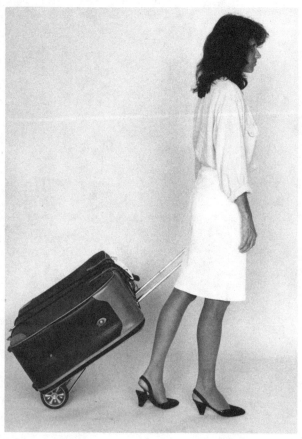

The Pain of Baggage Handling

Carrying heavy suitcases, brief cases, or grocery bags can produce neck, shoulder, arm, and back problems. This is more common than you might think. The stretching and imbalance, particularly if you carry weight on one side, can set off chronic pain. Many a traveler arrives home with lasting damage after having carried a heavy bag, using mainly one arm or only one side. Purchase a suitcase "jockey" on which you can wheel your luggage. These devices can accommodate almost any size bag. If you feel particularly flush, you can call for a porter.

I know many readers have the type of suitcase or luggage with wheels built into the bottom of the unit. These are satisfactory if they are pulled with a strap or some other device so that the stress is not placed on one side of the body. Using the luggage handle to propel the bag forward is not the proper way to do it.

Again, the point is to always remember to use both sides of your body, where possible, for any type of activity. For example, students who carry a large number of books should use a "knapsack" or "daypack." The weight distribution is over both shoulders—a much better way.

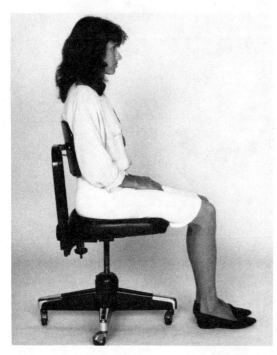

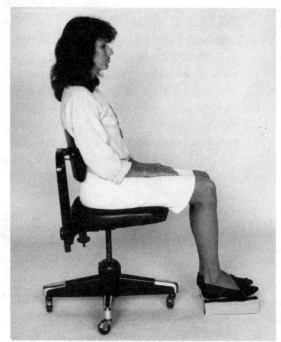

Sitting Pretty—and Pain Free

Office chairs are contributing to a nationwide backache among office workers. Most chairs have little more than a cushioned pad for mid-back support. That is not enough! You need a chair that can be adjusted to the person's individual height, and also to the unique contour and curve of his or her lower back.

If the company you work for won't seat you properly, you would be well advised to buy a folding orthopedic seat that is form-fitting and that provides good total support for your back. Such seats, obtainable at any good orthopedic supply shop, can be shaped by shop personnel to your proper fit.

Such seats have many uses. They can be used to make any other seat, including airline seats, theatre seats, or restaurant seats, into "good seats." More and more people are carrying their folded orthopedic seats under their arms to places where poor seating might otherwise inflict back pain.

When you are seated, never put your feet straight down to the floor. This transmits stress to the lower back. Instead, place something on the floor, like a telephone book (the Yellow Pages will do very well), under your feet. This will elevate your knees and take the stress off the knee areas. The back curve will be reduced, and you will have increased comfort.

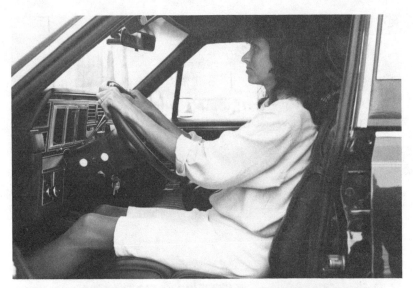

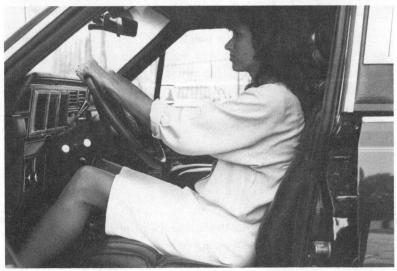

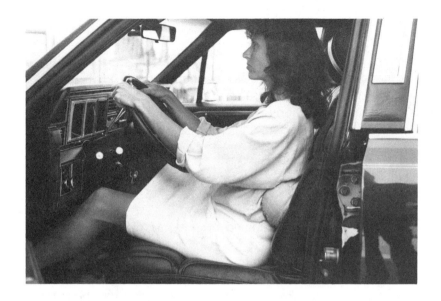

Car Seats—a Chronic Pain

While we are on the subject of seats, one of the most common sources of chronic pain in this country today is the automobile. Most of us spend many hours in our cars every week, driving parkways or freeways. (A few of us, indeed, literally live in our cars.) Yet, how many of us really take care to protect ourselves against poor automobile seating? Very few, I'm afraid.

We can make even the worst automobile seat much better by doing a few simple things. For example, we can place a telephone book or similar object on the floor at our feet so that when we are standing still in traffic, we might place our feet on the object, thereby relieving some of the stress building up in our lower extremities, back, and neck.

We can place a small, rolled-up towel, or some type of pad in the curve of the low back to reduce much of the stress in that area. The folding orthopedic seat we mentioned above can be very helpful in making a car seat less injurious.

Most cars do not have contour seats for support of the low back. Even in those cars that have them, the contour frequently does not provide enough support for the low back and certainly will not allow for a break at the knees.

When driving long distances, it is important to stop from time to time, get out of the car, walk around it a few times, or (if you don't mind the stares), squat alongside the car for awhile, then continue driving. If you are suffering from chronic back pain, stopping *every half hour* is recommended; otherwise, every hour will do.

The World's Worst Seats

Contrary to all those airline advertisements, airline seats are literally a pain in the rear, the whole back, and all over. They are the world's worst seats, for the simple reason that they are so padded as to allow your bottom to slide backward, pushing your spine into a forward position. Many business persons who travel frequently on airlines suffer chronic back discomfort. Again, you can place a book, your airline bag, a pillow, or a blanket under your feet, helping to raise your knees, much as I have recommended for both the office and the automobile. In addition, try to place some soft object, such as a pillow or a blanket in a rolled up fashion, at the small of your back.

Even first-class seats are not safe. Rest assured that those who travel in coach should not envy those who travel up front just because they have a wider seat. The contouring of their seat is almost as bad as yours.

To help remedy the problem, it is advisable to get out of your seat at least once every half hour and stretch. This can be done standing alongside the seat. If your seat belt is fastened, you can perform some stretching exercises while seated. Many of the airlines provide a booklet describing such exercises, and you should not hesitate to ask for it.

Bend your head forward and down, between your knees, and hold the position for a few minutes. Then, raise your knees to your chest, one at a time, holding the position for a few moments. With these two exercises, you will relieve some of the muscle and ligament strain in the low back area.

If you are on a flight lasting for more than one hour, it is advisable to move all parts of your body every 30 minutes or so to maintain good circulation. Each year, I see many patients who have been in a stationary position on long intercontinental flights, who have developed various vascular problems because of the hours-long immobility. This can happen in younger individuals, but it mostly involves older persons.

Recently, a physician friend of mine, in his mid-fifties, completed a marathon and shortly thereafer took a long flight. Despite the fact that he is in excellent shape, he developed a dangerous blood clot in an artery in his thigh. Severe pain developed in the area, and he was hospitalized for some special surgery. The greater danger, however, was that the clot might have traveled, causing even more problems. Fortunately, the clot remained fairly localized, but he still suffers from the after-effects of that long airplane trip. I am sorry to say he will not be running marathons for a long time to come.

So, please remember to keep moving!

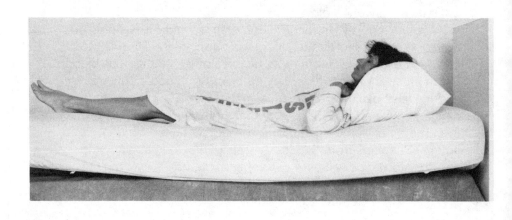

Don't Take Pain Lying Down

We spend about one-third of our lives in bed. Most of us would consider our bedroom a safe place, but this is not so. Beds, like people, age and sag in the middle. They develop mattress defects that can cause or aggravate back problems, as well as neck and shoulder problems. A sagging mattress is a bad mattress. A simple bed board, which can even be a large piece of plywood, placed between the mattress and the box spring is a good protection for your back. Firm mattresses are important. If you are using a waterbed, be sure the mattress is filled with water to the point where there is not too much "give."

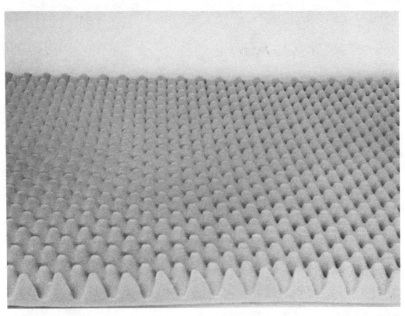

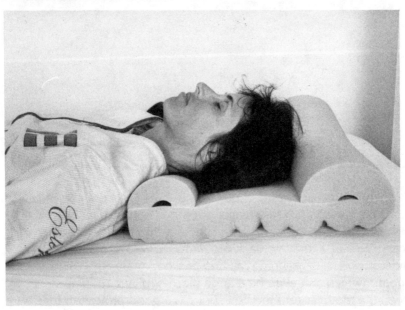

Aids to Pain-Free Sleeping

A very helpful bedroom item is the so-called "egg crate" mattress. If you have been hospitalized in recent years, you know that most hospitals on request will provide an egg crate mattress for their patients. These mattresses are not especially expensive. You can see why they call them "egg crate" mattresses by studying the photograph. Be a "good egg" and treat yourself right by getting one of these mattresses!

Several companies make cervical pillows that will support the curve in your neck while you sleep. Many options are available and we illustrate one of them. If you are handy, you can create your own pillow from some sponge rubber or cellulose padding. The main thing to remember is that you should feel a comfortable support at the curve of your neck. The pillow should be stabilized so that it does not slip away as you turn and twist during the night. These pillows now range in price from $25 to $50 at most department stores or sleep shops. Since we spend so much of our time in bed, all of us need this type of neck support.

My old grandmother's belief, "There is nothing like a good night's sleep to restore your energy and health," is as true today as when she declared it over 50 years ago. Look at your bed and make sure that it meets the minimum standards for proper rest. Ligaments and tendons, as well as bones, are put under a great deal of stress if your bed is defective.

Sleeping face down is not recommended for anyone, but if it is a necessity, at least place a small pillow under your abdomen so that the curve in your back is supported. The stress on your neck may be helped by proper pillow support. However, if you can retrain yourself, try to sleep either on your side or on your back.

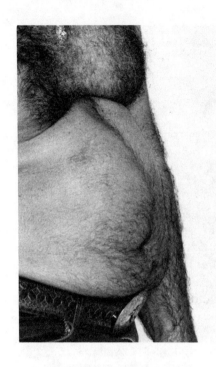

The Pains of Excess Weight: "Belly Blues!"

Overeating is not only bad for your figure, it can also bring on chronic pain, and I don't mean just a tummyache. Most Americans, even if they are in good shape, tend to have underdeveloped abdominal muscles because of excessive sitting, which we do daily, as well as because of our lack of exercise. Overeating causes a protrusion of the abdomen that many of us call a "pot belly." The belly sags forward, putting a powerful strain on the back. Obviously, a loss of weight is extremely important to anyone with back pain, or with any type of pain in the body, including the knees (which take a beating from the weight), as well as in the neck—which always suffers compensatory stress when the low back is involved.

The major problem of men over 40 (who tend to overeat and drink too much beer!) is chronic back pain. Usually, little can be done for such persons until they lose weight. Please read the chapters on weight control.

You should be sure to have your doctor's approval before you begin any exercise program. Given that, here are some exercises often used to "flatten your stomach."

To strengthen abdominal muscles, five minutes a day of bent knee sit-ups will help a lot. Be very careful when you start. Leg raises are also excellent for strengthening abdominal and back muscles. You should lie on your back, with a pillow under your head. Raise your legs slowly, keeping the knees straight, then slowly lower them to the count of 10. The effective movement is not as you are elevating the legs (in fact, you should not strain on doing so), but rather when slowly lowering them. This tends to strengthen the abdominal muscles. Remember that having strong abdominal muscles means that you have strong back muscles as well—there is a direct relation between these two muscle groups.

Never do sit-ups with straight legs since you have a good chance of severely hurting your back. Only the Rambo macho individuals among us should attempt this type of lethal activity. The stress placed on the intervertebral discs in the low back can frequently lead to a herniated nucleus pulposus ("ruptured" disc).

Intervertebral discs (they lie between the bony vertebrae of the spine), degenerate with the passage of time as they absorb the forces delivered daily to our body, and also as they become desiccated, or dried out, as part of the natural aging processes. A disc consists of a soft center surrounded by fibrous material. These fibers tend to fragment or separate as we grow older, and also as stress is placed on them. Sometimes the softer material inside will leak through to the outside. This may happen very rapidly, as when great forces are placed on the disc.

Performing such activities as straight-leg sit-ups, or other activities which raise the intradiscal pressure, can actually rupture the disc; the softer, inner material is rapidly extruded through a break in the fibrous "container." This may exert severely painful pressure against the spinal nerves, which branch out from the spine between the bony vertebral areas. At times, the "leak" is slow, and the pain develops in a slow but chronic fashion. Defects in the intervertebral discs are very common in all individuals. The problems become worse as one grows older, but they can exist in youngsters as well.

An important means of stabilizing the spine and preventing such problems is to have strong abdominal and spinal muscles. However, this must be achieved slowly over a period of many months, and the activity to strengthen these muscles should not be done rapidly. The sedentary lifestyle which most Americans enjoy today leads to a weakness in these discal areas.

A certain amount of physical activity, commonly called *exercise,* can be helpful in maintaining the integrity of the intervertebral areas. Rhythmic, gentle movement in the disc area, as well as

56

increased pumping of blood through the region by exercise, helps to maintain a youthful and structurally sound disc.

One of the objections I have to the mechanical exercise equipment used in many gyms and health clubs is that it can bring great force to bear on the delicate discal areas, particularly in the low back but also in the neck. If the exercise instructor is not properly trained or does not understand these problems, he or she may actually aggravate an underlying structural impairment, or may bring on a new problem by allowing unacceptable torsion or torque forces to be brought to bear on the back and neck. Therefore, you must be careful to guard yourself and get proper professional advice.

Sports physicians are seeing many more cases which have been brought about by mechanical exercise instruments that are used to strengthen muscles. If such physicians and allied health personnel derive a substantial portion of their living from the improper use of such equipment, why help them along? It is best to avoid use of such equipment until you have exercised to a point where your body is in good shape. A sagging abdomen or pot belly is a red flag against using this type of apparatus. Only abdominal and back muscles that are *already strong* will allow you to use this type of equipment safely.

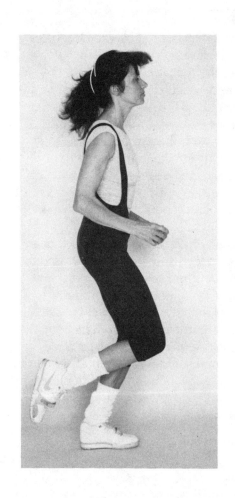

Exercise for Pain Prevention

I have left my most effective advice for the prevention of chronic pain for the last. Unless one undertakes an effective exercise program, he is almost certain to develop a chronic pain problem sometime during his lifetime. This has been demonstrated again and again as I have watched patients over the last 40 years.

An effective exercise program does not have to be of the strenuous type, which often scares people away from any type of leisure physical activity. I am talking about such things as doing aerobic exercise, which is fun and which can keep your muscles in good order with as little as 30 mintues exercise every other day.

I will not go into great detail on exercise, since I have co-authored a book which covers the topic intensively *(Going the Distance: The Right Way to Exercise for People Over 40),* listed at the back of this book. However, I want to stress the importance of exercise for the prevention of chronic pain problems and also for the treatment and control of chronic pain—rather than to talk about its merits in prolonging life or enhancing the quality of life. We know that exercise will help your heart, lungs, and blood vessels, but this is not what I am most concerned about in this book. Here, I stress the importance of exercise *to prevent chronic pain.*

Simply stated, *once your doctor says it is all right for you to exercise,* your exercise should be performed three times weekly, with a 10-minute warm-up period and a 10-minute warm-down period. The exercise should last for 30 minutes and make you perspire in a gentle fashion. It should be done continuously—without stopping—and in a rhythmic fashion, using all of the large muscles in the upper and lower part of your body. You should be *slightly* breathless only, and be able to carry on a conversation while you are exercising. The best exercise for most of us is walking. Certainly, it is the cheapest form of exercise and the least cumbersome.

Exercise increases circulation, strengthens muscles, and pumps important lymphatic fluid through the involved areas. Since most of our chronic pain develops in the back, neck, and knee areas, it is important to keep those areas in good condition. Simple exercise answers that need. Aerobic exercises, such as swimming, bicycling, walking, rowing, or cross-country skiing are recommended for the majority of us. Many of these exercises can be simulated indoors with home equipment, which is readily available and comparatively inexpensive. Exercise can be fun. I recommend to you not only my book but also many other exercise books at your library.

Suffice it to say, without some kind of exercise, you can look forward to developing a chronic pain problem. The human body was made to move and to have a certain amount of vigorous activity at frequent intervals. The nature of our life today—living in automobiles, sitting at desks, overeating, and over-indulging in many ways—clearly leads to the development of chronic pain syndromes.

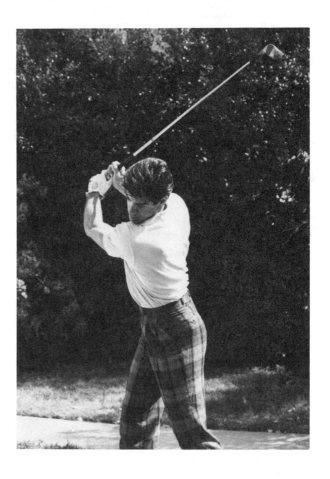

Balanced Exercise

Unfortunately, some of our leisure-time activities may also promote degenerative conditions in the back, neck, and various joint areas. Unilateral sports, such as golf, racquetball, and tennis frequently lead to stress in areas where we would not like to see such microtrauma. Rotation of an unstable back, as when swinging a golf club, as many of you well know, leads to pain in the low back area. The same is true of any of the other unilateral exercises. Bilateral exercises, utilizing both sides of the body, are much better. If you stay in good shape by consistent aerobic exercise of some type, the unilateral stress forces of golf, tennis, or racquetball will not produce the injuries they would otherwise.

Note the photograph of the golfer swinging the club. The torque forces produce changes in the neck and especially in the low back. The very folds of his shirt show the stress being transmitted to one side of the low back area. This happens every time you swing the golf club.

Part II

Weight Control for Pain Control

Weight Control with the CICO Diet: a Way to Control Appetite and Lose Weight

I am giving you the information in this chapter because I have learned that many of my patients have to lose weight for effective management of chronic pain problems. Most chronic pain problems are isolated to the low back area. More than 50 percent of patients presenting with chronic pain have pain in the low back, and many of these patients are overweight. These persons must lose weight in order to control their low back problems.

In addition, pain problems relating to the legs, the upper back, and the neck frequently are aggravated or perpetuated by excess weight. That is why I have had to take an interest in weight reduction problems.

In more than 40 years of practice, I have had the opportunity to study many patients who have been counselled by other physicians and weight reduction specialists. Thus, I have had the opportunity to study first hand various methods used to help patients lose weight. It has always troubled me that these methods have usually been very complex, and that many of them require the taking of harmful drugs or receiving equally harmful injections.

For many years of my practice, I was associated with a multi-specialty medical clinic. One of the physicians in that clinic, now deceased, was intensely interested in weight reduction problems. He devoted a great deal of time to researching the matter, and he was kind enough to convey his feelings and thoughts to me. Much of what he said can be readily appreciated, and it has been incorporated in this chapter. It gave him sheer joy to see a patient lose weight, and I must say that I feel the same exhilaration when I see a patient with chronic pain lose enough weight to relieve the problem. Of course, weight reduction is only one phase of chronic pain control, but, nevertheless, it is an important one—particularly with low back pain.

In telling patients how to lose weight, I had always been frustrated by the need to keep it as simple as possible and yet present as effective a plan as possible. So I decided many years ago to condense the information so that it could be presented very rapidly, even in just a few minutes. Essentially, that is what I am going to do in this short chapter and in the next chapter. I am not going to inundate you with information and a complex diet plan requiring special formulas. I am especially going to avoid recommending protein supplement diets—they make the cost and risk of weight reduction extreme. I am sure these protein diets can be effective, especially when used under medical supervision. However, we all know of the deaths and disabilities associated with some of these protein diets. In my view, they are an extreme approach to weight reduction. The basic concepts of healthful weight control have essentially been lost or clouded.

The CICO Formula

All diets should be based on a simple formula which is known and understood by all physicians and exercise physiologists. I am presenting what is called the CICO formula. The abbreviation CICO stands for Calories In, Calories Out. This very simple formula embodies the core or essence of all effective and safe weight reduction. Once a person settles on the type of exercise he will do on an every-other-day basis, the caloric load can be easily computed, and does not have to be done more than one time. I'll include some information on that in the next chapter.

Vitamin C and Appetite Suppression

One of the major challenges facing a person in trying to lose weight is the suppression of appetite. Any type of medication or pill which suppresses your appetite will often be either dangerous to use for long periods of time, or it will lose its effectiveness within a few short weeks. It is for this reason that I started to experiment with the commonly used vitamin C.

Perhaps one of the most unusual things about the CICO diet is its emphasis on vitamin C and the use of this naturally occurring substance to help control the appetite. Vitamin C is readily available and quite safe when used as directed. Some individuals may not be able to take this natural substance, but the principle of CICO still applies. Most individuals will be able to use vitamin C to control the appetite, and you should ask your doctor to be sure that you can use it. During the several decades I have been recommending this method, I have not found any patients who have suffered side effects which would be considered dangerous or who suffered side effects severe enough to discontinue using vitamin C. Some patients had to reduce the dose because they developed a slight diarrhea but after a dose reduction, they continued to use the vitamin. Nevertheless, you should ask your own doctor to be sure.

The appetite suppressant effect of Vitamin C is based on the fact that, when used a little while before meals, it will help to reduce the feeling of hunger by creating a counter feeling of fullness in the stomach and also a feeling of hunger satisfaction, or satiety. Your hunger pains can thus be controlled in what I believe is a safe manner for most people. In addition, you have the advantage that vitamin C is a healthful substance that is now commonly understood to improve the tissue integrity as well. Many even claim that it helps to reduce colds or upper respiratory infections. So much the better!

Therefore, the CICO formula not only reminds you to count the *Calories In* and the *Calories Out,* but also reminds you of the *vitamin C intake,* as well as the *vitamin C outgo.* (One reason vitamin C is generally so safe is that it is water soluble and readily excreted from the system.) Thus, for those who do not have an allergy or other special reaction to vitamin C, it makes a useful appetite suppressant. Again, most of my patients have had absolutely no side effects or difficulty with vitamin C, as we recommend using it, but you should have your own doctor's approval of this or any other health-related procedure.

How to Use the CICO Appetite Suppressant

One half hour before your planned meal, you should drink 8 ounces of the vitamin C mixture which I will recommend. It is better to prepare the mixture in advance and keep it refrigerated, or at least at a cool temperature, until you need it. Dissolve one teaspoon of powdered vitamin C (which usually contains 5,000 milligrams or 5 grams of ascorbic acid) in 16 ounces of water (one pint). The liquid is fairly stable (especially if kept in a refrigerator or in a cool area) and can, therefore, be prepared 24 or 48 hours in advance of the time you need it. If you wish to make a full quart of the mixture at one time, then you should use two teaspoons of the powdered vitamin C. Shake the mixture well, not only at the time you make it but also just before you use it. If you wish to use any other type of flavoring in the mixture, you can. I have used a small amount of condensed lemon juice or fresh lemon or lime juice in the fluid to give it additional flavor. You can also use a sugar substitute to sweeten the mixture, but, obviously, you want to avoid the actual use of sugar since this would add calories to the drink. I also do not recommend the use of fructose, since calories eventually are absorbed from fructose and do add to your daily caloric load, which you are trying to "keep down."

In summary, you simply take 8 fluid ounces of this vitamin C mixture one half hour before meals. You may wish to take more if you can tolerate it. You will find that there is a noticeable suppression of your appetite, which allows you to be satisfied with smaller portions of food, thus helping to prevent overeating.

A Continuing Metabolic Effect

The CICO formula can work wonders for you in a relatively short period of time, especially if you combine it with the exercise program I recommend. If you exercise every other day for at least 30 minutes, you will find that your basal metabolic rate will rise by a minimum of 10 percent, which will help you burn off more calories as the day goes on. Certainly, for at least one to two hours after you have completed exercises, you will continue to have the calorie-burning benefits of such exercise. It has been proven over and over again that exercise is one of the most effective ways to take off weight. This is especially true if your caloric load is held steady or if your caloric load is reduced to the basic calorie needs of your body.

Weight Control (and Pain Control) with Good Nutrition

We've talked about the way excess weight aggravates (and creates) pain problems and the urgent necessity to bring weight under control in order to bring pain under control. But where to go for good advice?

Each year several new diet books are published; in fact, some years see the birth of so many that if you lost ten calories in following the advice of each one you would easily achieve your ideal weight in no time. Unfortunately, most such books don't give you the effective method you need to control that adipose! *There are no real shortcuts* to a svelte figure. The CICO Plan, in the preceding chapter, is based on the simple reality that calorie expenditure is the name of the game.

Balance is Important

In constructing an effective diet, however, you must also construct a balanced diet. This balance depends upon having adequate protein, fats, and carbohydrates on your daily menu. Until recently, the accepted balance was 30 percent of caloric requirements in fat, 30 percent in protein, and the remainder in carbohydrates. However, in recent years dietitians and food scientists, backed by intensive research, have recommended that fats and protein should comprise only 20 percent each, and carbohydrates should be increased to 60 percent.

These recommendations are based on the fact that fats, especially cholesterol, could lead to hardening of the arteries, which could result in more heart attacks and strokes. Too much protein was considered unnecessary and perhaps harmful. The carbohydrates ideally should consist mainly of complex carbohydrates such as those in pasta, potatoes, fruits, vegetables, and so forth.

Simply then, you can divide your daily diet into 20 percent protein, 20 percent fat, and 60 percent carbohydrate, preferably complex carbohydrate. This will not only allow you to control your weight but also to reduce the possibility of disease development. There are no magic answers but this diet combined with exercise will offer you not only effective weight reduction but also *reduction of pain.*

Simple Calorie Counting

To determine the number of calories you need daily, proceed as follows. *Select your ideal weight,* which can be determined by asking your doctor or from insurance company charts showing ideal weight according to the type of frame you have (large, medium, or small). Take that figure (for example 154 pounds) and *divide by 2.2 pounds* (one kilogram) to determine your weight *in kilograms.*

In our example you would divide 154 by 2.2 to obtain 70 kilograms. *Multiply this figure by 24* (hours in a day) and you get 1680 calories. Finally, *determine your activity level* (which we hope will be greater than sedentary) according to your exercise and working habits.

For a sedentary person add 20 percent calories, for light activity add 30 percent, for moderate activity add 40 percent, and finally for vigorous daily activity add 50 percent.

In our example, if the 154 pound (70 kilogram) subject did light exercise (such as walking for 30 minutes a day) we would multiply 1680 by .30 to obtain an extra 404 calories which we add to 1680 and this equals 2084 calories. This then would be the number of calories you would need to reach your ideal weight or to maintain your ideal weight if you weighed 154 pounds and exercised or worked at a light level of activity.

To summarize, you take your weight in pounds, convert to kilograms, multiply by 24, and add a percentage according to your activity level.

Now you take the final figure and divide the caloric load into protein, fat, and carbohydrate needed on a 20, 20, 60 basis. In our example, the 2084 calories represents 417 calories each of protein and fat, at 20 percent each, while the remaining 60 percent, or 1250 calories, would go into carbohydrate.

Not So Fast

Please do not attempt to lose more than one to two pounds a week since that is a reasonable, healthy goal. To do this you would approach your ideal caloric goal (if you are overweight) by reducing your daily caloric load by about 500 calories per day if you want to lose about one pound a week—up to 1000 calories per day to lose two pounds a week. Remember, though, not to lower your daily intake below 1,200 calories per day under any circumstances. To do so might be inadvisable and hard on your body.

Choose your protein carefully since the quality of your protein does matter in maintaining health. If you use meat, fish and fowl are better than beef, especially if the beef contains a lot of fat. The old marbled steak is out, but a serving of lean beef can be taken once or twice a week. Vegetables and legumes, such as soy beans, are an excellent source of protein. Beef contains a high proportion of animal cholesterol, which can lead to hardening of the arteries, which in turn can lead to a propensity toward heart attacks and strokes. Vegetable sources of cholesterol do not cause these same problems.

Fats Are Important

Fats are indeed necessary to maintain life. Many of our hormones need fat in order to be synthesized, while the vital lining around many nerves requires fat in its manufacture. Twenty percent fat in our diets is a reasonable amount. Some diet plans which have become popular in recent years recommend even less than 20 percent, while the American Heart Association has reduced its recommended levels of fat to below 30 percent in most instances.

The present belief, held by most food scientists, is that this fat would best be in the polyunsaturated or monounsaturated categories. Polyunsaturated fats include corn, soy, and safflower oils while monounsaturated fats include olive oil and canola oils as well as peanut oil. Olive oil appears to be more accepted at present; peanut oil is still up for judgment. Recent research seems to indicate that monounsaturated oils are the best to use in the prevention of hardening of the arteries—better than even polyunsaturates.

Don't Eliminate Fats

You should reduce saturated fats in your diet where possible, but you don't have to eliminate them. Butter, lard, animal fats (as in beef), all comprise this category. You can use butter, but sparingly. Avoid coconut and palm oils if you can. I know it is hard to do since so many processed food products contain them. However, in future years you are going to see less and less of them in the ingredients listed on food packages. Coconut and palm oils lead to marked elevation of cholesterol, particularly the bad fraction of cholesterol, LDL, or the low density type. The high density lipids (fats) known as HDL cholesterol are the kind of friends you want. HDL fats lead to less arterial hardening and thus help to reduce the likelihood of strokes and heart attacks. Exercise and proper diet lead to an elevation of HDL and a reduction of the unfavorable LDL fraction.

Carbohydrates Are Crucial

Carbohydrates, particularly complex carbohydrates, are all the rage now and for good reason. Foods such as whole grains, nuts, vegetables, particularly legumes like beans, not only supply us with sustaining sources of energy but also add necessary fiber to our diets. The starches in complex carbohydrates give us a source of energy which is unparalleled. Complex carbohydrates break down more slowly than do simple sugars and thereby give a more sustained source of energy to the body. Although simple sugars, such as those from cane sugar, and contained in candy, can supply quick energy.

More effective longer term energy requirements are better met by complex carbohydrates. Simple sugar, in my experience, can many times make a chronic pain problem worse. You may hurt more after ingesting such a sugar. The mechanism seems to relate

72

to the effect of sugar on calcium metabolism and calcium plays a major role in pain transmission. Many of my arthritic patients note more pain developing after simple sugar intake.

A Sweet Treat

Incidentally, if you crave a sweet-tasting drink which won't add many calories to your diet and which can usually satisfy your appetitie, try this suggestion which has worked so well for my patients. Add a teaspoon or two teaspoons of powdered dry milk (skim or low fat milk) to a glass (8 to 10 ounces) of a diet beverage, (such as a cola) and, voilà, you have a bubbly drink which tastes like an ice-cream soda and looks like one but without the calories or sugar. Incidentally, a nice side effect of this creation is that it fills your tummy and reduces your appetitie. If you take it a half hour before meals it can keep down your hunger pangs and help to reduce your food intake if that is what you need to do. It works well with the vitamin C I recommended on the CICO Plan.

Fiber, The Great Cleanser

Dietary fiber is vital to not only your digestion but also to help reduce that notorious cholesterol level. We now know for sure that a certain amount of fiber in your diet is necessary to reduce your risk of bowel cancer. Those who do not include adequate fiber in their daily menu have a markedly increased chance of getting an intestinal carcinoma in later life.

Fiber also helps to flush out cholesterol. Many of the complex carbohydrates contain wonderful sources of fiber. Vegetables, fruits, and grains have a fibrous structure. The current popularity of oat bran to help lower cholesterol levels is well founded. Other brans such as wheat bran can do the same, but ounce for ounce, oat bran works somewhat better. Brans and many of the complex carbohydrates also contain silicon which is important in bone formation and membrane integrity, and therefore can help in certain painful conditions such as arthritis.

Fluids Ease Pain

Please remember to get adequate fluids, particularly water, into your daily routine. Pain problems are all made worse when a patient is dehydrated or has an inadequate body fluid level. I recommend at least eight ounces of fluid to be ingested for each waking hour. For example, if you are up 16 hours a day, I feel that you should get at least 128 ounces of fluid, or eight to nine pints per day. I realize that this may be hard for the average person to do, but you can increase your intake in relation to meal times and before and after exercise. The CICO Diet works better with proper fluid intake. For those who find that taking fluids just before sleep or within a few hours before sleep results in their having to arise frequently at night can increase their intake during the earlier hours of the day. Remember, fluid (and water is the best) not only helps to lubricate the joints but also keeps skin looking young and the bowels functioning better.

To Supplement or Not?

What about vitamin and mineral supplements, are they necessary and, if so, how much? Well, if you follow the balanced diet I have recommended, supplementation may not be absolutely necessary. However, in today's world of stress and exposure to toxic pollutants, some vitamin and mineral supplementation seems advisable, especially for pain prevention and control.

Vitamins

I usually recommend a so-called B-100 vitamin formula which can be obtained at your local health food store or pharmacy. This combination of B vitamins (B-complex) offers a simple, single dose of adequate level for anyone. It's true that B vitamins are water soluble, and you may urinate out a fair portion of the vitamins, but your body will retain what it needs, especially if a deficient condition exists. Also, B vitamins are needed in combination with amino acids (which are derived from protein) to produce certain neurotransmitters necessary for pain control. For example, B_6 works well with tryptophan (an amino acid) to help produce serotonin, a neurotransmitter vitally concerned with pain reduction. So the B-100 formula seems to help do the trick.

As to vitamin C, the CICO Diet plan will give you an adequate amount in most instances. I usually prefer that a pain patient ingest between 2000 to 3000 milligrams (or 2 to 3 gms) of vitamin C a day—if the person has no problem with the vitamin. Some individuals have diarrhea or an aggravation of gouty arthritis, when using large amounts of vitamin C. Most, however, can easily handle this amount of vitamin C I have recommended. Vitamin C is important in tissue oxygenation, and the amount of oxygen in your body tissues is important in pain control. Impaired cellular oxygen levels can increase painful conditions.

The fat-soluble vitamins, A, D, E, and K, are adequately provided in most cases by the type and level of fat ingestion recommended above. Some scientists now feel that we should supplement our vitamin E intake since it has a very important role in nervous system physiology and cell membrane integrity. Personally, I recommend taking 400 to 800 mgs of vitamin E a day. The questions about vitamin E might fill a book in itself, but, suffice it to say, 400 to 800 mgs a day can't hurt and may help pain patients while the jury is still out, and before a final verdict is rendered.

Minerals

Mineral supplementation seems vital in a few areas. One important situation involves women and calcium intake. I strongly urge all women to take 1500 milligrams of calcium daily along with 1000 milligrams of magnesium. It is true that many physicians recommend that post menopausal women take this amount and recommend slightly less for younger women, *but* the 1500 milligram calcium and 1000 milligram magnesium supplementation is fine and, frankly, much easier to remember for lifetime usage.

Calcium and magnesium must be taken for life, and studies during the last decade show that women should start the supplementation as early as menarche (age 14 or 15) in order to prevent osteoporosis, or thinning of bones, in later life. Exercise, calcium, and adequate female hormone levels can markedly reduce and even eliminate osteoporosis if begun early enough. Osteoporosis is a common cause of spinal pain in older women, and control of this problem should start as early as the teen years. See your doctor for further details on this important matter. Here is a definite situation where a stitch in time saves nine.

When selecting your calcium be careful to check the label on the bottle to see that the preparation contains 1500 milligrams of *elemental calcium.* If so, that is the actual amount of calcium your body is receiving. Often the calcium is given as higher than the elemental level, but you are only receiving the amount of elemental calcium listed. Calcium carbonate is the least expensive and the most satisfactory type. This is the kind contained in oyster shells and in some antacid tablets. These antacids make for an excellent, inexpensive source of calcium. However, check the label carefully!

Other minerals are also important in dealing with pain problems.

Zinc, for example, is a versatile and vital trace mineral that is an essential part of more than 70 enzyme systems. These systems control growth, healing, and maintenance of skin, hair, nails, and mucous membrane. Since many pain problems are due to inflammation of body tissues, zinc is important in the healing process. Also, under stress and during strenuous exercise, zinc is lost from the body. Recent research shows that, with exercise, zinc is lost in sweat and urine—even more with strenuous exercise. Following extended, strenuous exercise and prolonged, heavy perspiration, zinc loss can exceed 20 percent of the recommended daily allowance (RDA). Zinc is contained in foods such as oysters, liver, dark meat from chicken and turkey, and other high-protein foods. However, with my chronic pain patients I recommend taking 15 milligrams to 25 milligrams daily as a supplement.

Still other minerals may play a role in pain problems or in pain control. However, at this time the evidence for their usage on a daily basis is not clear enough for me to recommend them as supplements to your diet. Certainly, there would be no harm in adding a one-a-day mineral formula to your regimen. Many health food stores and pharmacies offer such a single multi-mineral tablet or capsule. Just remember to read the labels carefully so that you know what you are getting.

Average Calories Expended in Various Activities

(These are approximate average values for someone weighing 140–150 lbs. They include the energy needed for basal metabolism.)

Activity		Calories Per:		
		Hour	Half-hour	Minute
Sleeping (for comparison)		75	38	1.25
RECREATION AND EXERCISE				
Walking on level	2.0 mph	180	90	3.00
	3.0 mph	260	130	4.33
	3.5 mph	300	150	5.00
	4.0 mph	350	175	5.83
	4.5 mph	480	240	8.00
	5.3 mph	620	310	10.33
Walking upstairs	1.0 mph	195	98	3.25
	2.0 mph	640	320	10.67
Walking downstairs	2.0 mph	215	108	3.58
Running on level	5.5 mph	660	330	11.00
	7.2 mph	720	360	12.00
	8.0 mph	825	413	13.75
	10.0 mph	1140	570	19.00
	11.4 mph	1390	695	23.17
Hiking (20-lb. pack)	2.5 mph	300	150	5.00
	3.0 mph	312	156	5.20
	3.5 mph	380	190	6.33
	4.0 mph	450	225	7.50

From: *The Complete Guide to Physical Fitness,* courtesy of Authors Paul J. Kiell, M.D., and Joseph Frelinghuysen; and Publisher Stephen Glick, Stoeger Publishing Company, South Hackensack, NJ 07606.

Activity		Calories Per:		
		Hour	Half-hour	Minute
Hiking (40-lb. pack)	1.0 mph	210	105	3.50
	2.0 mph	270	135	4.50
	3.0 mph	348	174	5.80
	4.0 mph	540	270	9.00
Swimming				
Crawl stroke	0.7 mph	300	150	5.00
	1.0 mph	420	210	7.00
	1.6 mph	700	350	11.67
	1.9 mph	850	425	14.17
	2.2 mph	1600	800	26.67
Breast stroke	0.7 mph	300	150	5.00
	1.0 mph	410	205	6.83
	1.3 mph	600	300	10.00
Side stroke	1.0 mph	550	275	9.17
	1.6 mph	1200	600	20.00
Back Stroke	0.8 mph	300	150	5.00
	1.0 mph	450	225	7.50
	1.2 mph	540	270	9.00
	1.33 mph	660	330	11.00
	1.6 mph	800	400	13.33
Bicycling	5.5 mph	240	120	4.00
	9.0 mph	415	208	6.92
	13.0 mph	660	330	11.00
Skiing				
On level	3.0 mph	540	270	9.00
	5.0 mph	720	360	12.00
Downhill	Various	300–500	150–250	5.0–8.33
Skating	Leisurely	350	175	5.83
	9.0 mph	470	235	7.83
	11.0 mph	640	320	10.67
	13.0 mph	780	390	13.00
Snowshoeing	2.5 mph	620	310	10.33
Rowing	2.5 mph	300	150	5.00
	3.5 mph	660	330	11.00
	11.0 mph	970	485	16.17

Activity		Calories Per:		
		Hour	Half-hour	Minute
Canoeing	Leisurely	230	115	3.83
	4.0 mph	420	210	7.00
Baseball				
(Except pitcher)		300	150	5.00
Pitcher		400	200	6.67
Volleyball				
Recreational		350	175	5.83
Competitive		600	300	10.00
Basketball		608	304	10.13
Tennis				
Recreational		450	225	7.50
Competitive and singles		600	300	10.00
Golf (no carts)		300	150	5.00
Bowling		270	135	4.50
Squash		600–800	300–400	10.00–13.33
Fencing		630	315	10.50
Horseback riding (trot)		415	208	6.92
Badminton				
Recreational		350	175	5.83
Competitive		600	300	10.00
Mountain climbing		600	300	10.00
Table tennis		360	180	6.00
GENERAL FITNESS EXERCISES				
Basic level		200	100	3.33
Intermediate and advanced levels		400	200	6.67
GENERAL				
Lying down		85	43	1.42
Watching TV in chair		107	54	1.78
Mental work (seated)		110	55	1.83
Sewing, handwork		115	58	1.92
Dressing and undressing		140	70	2.33
Driving a car		150	75	2.50

Activity	Calories Per:		
	Hour	Half-hour	Minute
Office work	155	78	2.58
Light housework	165	83	2.75
Ironing	150	75	2.50
Sweeping, vacuuming	180	90	3.00
Cleaning windows	195	98	3.25
Polishing	210	105	3.50
Laundry work	240	120	4.00
Making beds	270	135	4.50
Mopping	300	150	5.00
Gardening	250	125	4.17
House painting	225	113	3.75
Chopping wood	480	240	8.00
Sawing wood	515	258	8.58
Stacking firewood	370	185	6.17
Carpentry work	230	115	3.83
Shoveling dirt	425	213	7.08
Stone masonry	420	210	7.00
Machinist work (light)	180	90	3.00
Printing work	150	75	2.50

Say, "Goodbye Pain!"

I do hope the information in this book helps you to prevent chronic pain problems. Eighty percent of these problems can and will be avoided or stopped by following the guidelines I have given. The other 20 percent develop from accidental injuries which cannot be controlled, and from conditions with which a person is born, amplified over the years.

Since most of the pain problems we all have involve the low back and neck area, and headaches, you can readily see that such problems are likely to be self-induced in approximately 80 percent of all cases. If you heed my advice, you will enjoy as many pain-free years of life as can possibly be obtained with rational living. You can, indeed, say "Goodbye Pain!"

Other Books by Dr. Lawrence:

Going the Distance: the Right Way to Exercise for People Over 40 (with Sandra Rosenzweig), Los Angeles, CA: Jeremy P. Tarcher, 1987. (May be ordered directly from Dr. Ronald M. Lawrence, 28240 Agoura Rd., Suite 202, Agoura Hills, CA 91301, at $15.95, postpaid.)

Pain Relief with Osteomassage (with Stanley Rosenberg), Santa Barbara, CA: Woodbridge Press, 1982, $5.95, postpaid.